DIABETES RECIPES COOKBOOK

"Delicious and Nutritious: A Diabetes-Friendly Culinary Journey"

Lorri Lazini

COPYRIGHT

CONTENTS

INTRODUCTION

Diabetes mellitus ("diabetes mellitus") is a serious disease that occurs when the body has difficulty properly regulating the amount of dissolved sugar (glucose) in the blood. It has nothing to do with diabetesinsipidus, a disease of the same name that causes problems with water retention in the kidneys. To understand diabetes, you must first understand the role of glucose in the body and what happens when glucose levels become uncontrolled and blood sugar levels become dangerously low or high. The tissues and cells that make up the human body are living organisms and require nutrients to survive.

The food absorbed into cells is a type of sugar called glucose. Because the body's cells are stationary, glucose transport is entirely dependent on the bloodstream containing the cells. Without adequate access to glucose, the body's cells lack energy and quickly die. People eat foods that are not glucose. Human food is converted to glucose during normal digestion. After metabolism, glucose enters the blood and the concentration of dissolved glucose in the blood increases. The bloodstream then carries the dissolved glucose to various tissues and cells in the body.

Glucose is in the blood, but neighboring cells cannot access it without the help of a chemical hormone called insulin. Insulin acts as a key that unlocks the cells, allowing them to absorb and use available glucose. When insulin is present, cells absorb glucose from the blood, and as sugar leaves the blood and enters the cells, blood sugar levels drop. Insulin can be considered a glucose bridge between the blood and cells. It is important to understand that as insulin levels increase, blood sugar levels decrease (sugar enters the cells and is used for energy). The body is designed to regulate and buffer the amount of dissolved glucose in the blood, maintaining a continuous supply of glucose to meet cellular needs.

The pancreas, one of many organs in the body, produces and stores insulin, then releases it into the blood to lower blood sugar levels. The concentration of glucose available in the blood at any given time depends on the amount and type of food a person eats. Refined carbohydrates, cookies, and candies are easily broken down into glucose. Therefore, eating these foods causes your blood sugar levels to spike. Conversely, after consuming more complex unrefined carbohydrates (e.g. oatmeal, apples, baked potatoes), blood sugar levels rise more gradually and slowly, requiring more digestion steps before they can be produced.

When blood sugar levels suddenly rise, your body must react quickly by immediately releasing large amounts of insulin. Otherwise, you risk developing a dangerous condition called hyperglycemia (hyperglycemia). We'll talk about this later. The influx of insulin delivers glucose into the cells and lowers glucose levels. While glucose levels rise and fall quickly, insulin levels change much more slowly.

When you eat large amounts of simple sugars, your blood quickly fills with glucose. Glucose enters the cells immediately, but high levels of insulin remain in the blood for some time. This can cause too much insulin in the blood, causing hunger and another serious condition called hypoglycemia (hypoglycemia). If blood sugar rises slowly, drastic adjustments are less necessary. Insulin is released in a controlled and safe manner, putting less stress on the body. This gradual process provides a sense of "satisfaction" or contentment over a long period of time.

For this reason, it is best for your overall health to limit the amount and frequency of sweets and refined sugars in your diet. Instead, eat more complex carbohydrates, such as fresh fruit, whole grain bread or pasta, and legumes. The difference between simple and complex sugars (carbohydrates) is likened to the difference between white bread (simple) and whole grain bread (more complex).

Insulin is a major key to the ability of cells to use glucose. If there is a problem with insulin production or how cells perceive insulin, the body's balanced glucose metabolism can easily spin out of control. When these problems occur, diabetes can occur, causing blood sugar levels to fluctuate and damaging the body.

Overview

Diabetes is a metabolic disorder that causes the body to convert food into energy. The body uses digestive juices to break down food into the energy components it needs to survive, including a sugar called glucose. After digestion, glucose enters the bloodstream and is absorbed and used by cells or stored for later use.

For cells to absorb glucose, a hormone called insulin must be present in the blood. Insulin acts as a "key" that opens the "door" on the cell surface and allows glucose to enter the cell. Special cells (islet cells) produce insulin in an organ called the pancreas, which is about 6 inches long and located behind the stomach. In people without diabetes, the pancreas automatically produces enough insulin to allow glucose to enter the cells. In people with diabetes, the body does not produce or use insulin properly. If glucose cannot enter the cells, it accumulates in the blood.

The buildup of glucose in the blood (sometimes called

hyperglycemia or hyperglycemia (meaning "too much glucose in the blood")) is a sign of diabetes. When blood sugar levels rise above a certain level, excess glucose leaks from the kidneys (organs that filter waste from the blood) into the urine. Glucose also absorbs water, causing frequent urination and thirst. These two symptoms, frequent urination and abnormal dry mouth, are often the first signs of diabetes. This often results in calories and water being lost through urine, resulting in weight loss. When the body stops producing insulin, it must receive insulin from another source: insulin injections or an insulin pump. If your body does not use insulin properly, you may be able to take oral medications as an alternative to or in addition to insulin injections.

However, neither insulin nor other drugs can cure diabetes. They simply help control the disease.

Effective Diabetes Management in Schools

A. Effective treatment of diabetes

The goal of effective diabetes treatment is to control blood sugar levels within the target range established for each child. Optimal glycemic control promotes normal growth and development and ensures optimal learning. Effective diabetes management is necessary to prevent the immediate risk of blood sugar levels being too high or too low. The key to optimal blood sugar control is a careful balance of diet, exercise, and insulin or medications. In general, food raises blood sugar, and exercise and insulin lower it. Blood sugar levels can also be affected by many other factors, such as growth and puberty, psychological stress, illness, or injury.

The key to optimal blood sugar control is a careful balance of diet, exercise, and insulin or medications.

Students with diabetes should monitor their blood sugar levels throughout the day using a glucometer. The device displays blood sugar levels when measured. If blood sugar levels are too low (hypoglycemia) or too high (hyperglycemia), students can take corrective action, such as changing their diet, activity level, or insulin use. The most immediate risk for people with diabetes is hypoglycemia, which in rare cases can be life-threatening.

Many students are able to manage all or most of their diabetes care on their own. Some children may require assistance from staff due to their age, level of development or lack of experience. The school nurse is the best person to care for students with diabetes in the school setting. But managing diabetes requires working 24 hours a day, 7 days a week, and diabetes emergencies can happen at any time. More importantly, the school nurse is not always present. Therefore, the school board must designate appropriate school personnel to respond to emergencies in the school and during school -sponsored activities involving students with diabetes. In this case, the school nurse must ensure adequate training of qualified school personnel and provide specialized supervision and guidance in routine and emergency care of the student.

B. Plan and implement effective diabetes management

Collaboration, collaboration and planning are key elements to successful diabetes management in schools. Like children with other chronic illnesses, students, parents, school nurses, principals, teachers, other school staff, and the student's health care provider (or care team) personal care) work together to achieve goals. , students with diabetes are also more likely to succeed in school. The goal is to provide effective diabetes treatment. Your local school district may have a similar plan or system for children with other medical conditions.

To work together, districts should form school teams of people knowledgeable about diabetes, school environments, and federal and state education and management laws. Team members may include students, parents, school nurses, school nutrition and other health care personnel, administrators, principals, teachers, counselors, and other relevant individuals. This team works together to implement recommendations from the student's personal and family health team. The team determines who will receive relevant medical information about the child and who will receive nursing training to help monitor and perform specific tasks.

Additionally, school teams should be part of the team that develops and implements educational needs to ensure that diabetes is managed safely and effectively in schools. The plan is based in part on the student's medical recommendations, also known as the Diabetes Medical Management Plan (DMMP), as well as the team's recommendations.

C. Federal and state laws

Many laws define school districts' obligations to accommodate students with diabetes on a case-by-case basis. Some federal laws require all schools that receive federal funds to provide appropriate consideration for the special needs of children with diabetes. If services are determined to be appropriate, federal law requires that a normal learning environment be maintained for the child to minimize disruption to the child's school and daily life while allowing the child to participate fully in all school activities. It requires personal judgment and reasonable accommodation within the company.

Schools are responsible for understanding all applicable federal and state laws and how they impact their policies.

Below is a brief description of the most important state and federal laws.

CGS 10-212a Medication Management in Schools. This law concerns drug use in schools. This law regulates who can prescribe medications and who can administer medications in schools. Connecticut State Agency Code Sections 10-212a-1 through 10-212a-10, Administration of Drugs by School Staff and Administration of Drugs in After-School and After-School Preparation Programs. These policies govern the procedural aspects of school drug administration.

Rules contain definitions within the rule. Components of local drug regulatory policy. Staff training. Self-administration of medications. Handling, storage and disposal of pharmaceutical products. Drug monitoring. Medication administration is administered by licensed athletic trainers and coaches at intramural and interscholastic events. Paraprofessional medication management and administration in preschool and after-school programs.

Public Bill 12-198 (HB 5348) A bill regarding the management of medications for students with diabetes, the role of school counselors, the availability of Board of Education CPR and AED information, and physical activity during the school day. This law allows the school nurse or a qualified school employee appointed by the principal to administer an emergency glucagon injection to a bleeding student under certain circumstances and with the consent of the student's parents and a prescription from the student's physician.

The bill also prohibits schools from restricting when and where a student with diabetes can test his blood sugar at school if he has the permission of his parents or guardian and a written order from a doctor. The bill expands school district guidelines on how to manage students with lifelong allergies to include students with glycogen storage disease. He wants the State Department of Education and

Health to issue new guidelines by July 1, 2012, and for school districts to improve self-treatment and glycogen deposition treatment for students with the disease, effective from the August 15, 2012 disease plan. The plan must allow the parent or guardian of the student with the disorder, or their representative, to provide food or nutrition to the student with the disorder at school during the school day.

The law prohibits claims against cities, school districts, and school officials for damages resulting from these actions. Section 504 of the Affordable Care Act of 1973 also protects the rights of children who are disabled and require reasonable assistance to receive a "free and appropriate public education" (FAPE). The law applies to all projects and activities that receive government funding, including public schools. If a child has a physical or mental disability that prevents him or her from performing basic life activities, he or she has the right to receive assistance under Section 504. Basic activities include walking, seeing, hearing, speaking, breathing, learning, working, personal care and physical activity.

It is often considered necessary because of the unique nutritional and metabolic needs of children with diabetes. Students do not need to receive special services to benefit from other services. The Individuals with Disabilities Education Act (IDEA) of 1976 provides financial assistance to state and local agencies for the education of students with disabilities. Children are eligible if they have one or more of 13 disability categories and need special education and related services due to their disability. Commonly used for children with diabetes are other health conditions (OHI). It is defined as "a lack of hypervigilance to the learning environment due to a lack of energy, strength, or alertness, including hyperalertness to environmental stimuli." 1) Sexual intercourse due to chronic or serious illness; 2) Negative impact on children's education. The Family Educational Rights and Privacy Act of 1974 (FERPA) protects the privacy of students and parents by limiting access to school records that contain private letters containing student information. The law sets standards for keeping student information confidential.

FERPA also establishes standards for informing parents and eligible students of their rights to access information and to control where and when that information may not be disclosed outside of school without permission. Special thoughts from parents. Under FERPA, schools are required to notify school officials if there is a legitimate educational interest. Connecticut public schools must meet standards set by the Occupational Safety and Health Administration (OSHA), the regulatory agency of the U.S. Department of Labor.

These standards include the need to have procedures to control potential exposure to blood-borne pathogens. OSHA regulations require schools to provide a clean and healthy learning environment. Schools all over the world need to be careful to protect themselves from the risk of blood-borne diseases. This includes the use of barriers such as surgical gloves and other protective measures when handling blood, other body fluids, and tissues. These federal laws provide a framework for planning and implementing effective diabetes care in schools. School administrators and parents should consider whether state or local laws should be considered when supporting students with diabetes.

D. School Schedule

 Schools are responsible for being familiar with all applicable federal and state laws and their impact on policy in this area. CSDE recommends that schools develop plans to address the health needs of children with diabetes. This plan should be based in part on the student's Medical Management Plan (also known as the Diabetes Medical Management Plan (DMMP)). The DMMP is completed by the student's parent/legal guardian and health care provider. This often includes   specific instructions for monitoring blood sugar levels, using insulin, and responding to emergency situations, as well as recognizing and treating hypoglycemia and hyperglycemia. A written diabetes education plan for each student helps students, families, staff, and health care providers know what to expect.

Once the team sets these expectations, they should put them in writing in the following documents: Individual Health Care Plan (IHCP) – The IHCP describes how the school intends to meet safety and health   requirements. Everyday health for everyone. School direction. control. The IHCP was developed by school nurses in collaboration with parents, students, health care providers, and other school staff. IHCPs typically serve students who have multiple health needs or who require daily intervention based on their health needs.

This plan includes a health assessment, nursing diagnosis, and review of goals and action plans that address a variety of potential problems. Emergency Care Plan (ECP) – The ECP is based on information provided by the student's health care providers, family, and school. The ECP explains how to recognize hypoglycemia and hyperglycemia and what to do if you notice signs and symptoms of these conditions. PCUs are often part of an IHCP.

An emergency plan provides specific instructions on what to do in an emergency. These written plans help nurses, school staff, and first responders respond quickly, safely, and independently to emergency situations. Education plan. This plan includes: Plans, such as Section 504 plans and Individualized Education Programs (IEPs), describe the accommodations, educational supports, and services needed for each student.

Body

Types of Diabetes

What are the types of diabetes?

The most common types of diabetes are type 1 diabetes, type 2 diabetes and gestational diabetes.

Type 1 Diabetes

If you have type 1 diabetes, your body produces little or no insulin. Type 1 diabetes is usually diagnosed in children and adults, but it can occur at any age.

Type 2 Diabetes

If you have type 2 diabetes, your body cannot use insulin properly. The pancreas produces insulin, but not enough insulin to keep blood sugar within the normal range. You may develop type 2 diabetes if you are at risk for being overweight or obese and the disease is genetic. You can slow or stop the development of type 2 diabetes by identifying risk factors and taking health measures such as weight loss or prevention.

Gestational Diabetes

Usually this type of diabetes disappears after the baby is born. However, if you have gestational diabetes, you may have a higher risk of developing type 2 diabetes in the future. A diagnosis of diabetes during pregnancy may be type 2 diabetes.

Prediabetes

People with pre-diabetes, blood sugar is higher than normal but not high enough to be diagnosed with type 2 diabetes. Having prediabetes increases your risk of developing type 2 diabetes in the future. They also have a higher risk of heart disease than people with normal diabetes. Other Types of Diabetes A rare type of diabetes called monogenic diabetes is caused by a mutation in a single gene.

Diabetes can also result from pancreatic surgery to remove the pancreas or from damage to the pancreas due to conditions such as cystic fibrosis (external link to pancreatic cancer), infection, and pancreatitis.

What about diabetes and pre-diabetes?

More than 133 million Americans have diabetes or prediabetes.

1. In 2019, 37.3 million people (11.3% of the American population) had diabetes. At least one in four people over the age of 65 has diabetes. Approximately one-third of adults with diabetes do not know they have diabetes.

2. Approximately 90-95% of diabetic patients have type 2 diabetes.

3. In 2019, 38% of American adults, or 96 million people, had prediabetes.

4. What other health problems can people with diabetes have? Over time, high blood sugar can cause damage to your heart, kidneys, legs, and eyes. If you have diabetes, you can take steps to reduce your risk of developing diabetes by improving your health and learning how to manage your condition. Controlling your blood sugar, blood pressure, and cholesterol levels can help prevent future health problems.

Diabetes symptoms

Diabetes symptoms are defined by high blood sugar levels. Some people, especially those with pre-diabetes, gestational diabetes, or type 2 diabetes, may have no symptoms. In the case of type 1 diabetes, symptoms appear quickly and often become more severe.

Symptoms

Feeling thirstier than usual and urinating frequently. Losing weight is easy. Ketone bodies are present in urine. Ketone bodies are formed due to the breakdown of muscle and fat that occurs when there is a lack of insulin. I feel tired and weak. Irritability and other mood changes. Blurred vision. Wounds heal gradually. Many infections occur, including gum infections, skin infections, and surgical infections. However, it often begins in childhood or adolescence. Type 2 diabetes, the most common type, can occur at any age.

Causes

To understand diabetes, it is important to understand how the body uses glucose correctly.

How does insulin work?

Insulin is a hormone produced by glands located behind and below the stomach (pancreas).

The pancreas releases insulin into the blood. Insulin circulates and allows sugar to enter cells. Insulin lowers blood sugar levels. As blood sugar levels drop, the amount of insulin secreted by the pancreas also decreases.

Effects of Glucose

Glucose (sugar) is a source of energy for the cells that make up muscles and other organs. Glucose comes from two main sources: food and the liver. Sugar is absorbed into the blood and enters cells through insulin. The liver stores and produces glucose. When blood sugar levels drop, such as when you have not eaten for a while, the liver breaks down stored glycogen into glucose.

This will keep your blood sugar levels at normal levels. The exact cause of various types of diabetes is not known. In both cases, sugar builds up in the blood. It is unclear what these factors are.

Risk Factors

Risk factors for developing diabetes depend on the type of diabetes. Family history can play a role in many ways. Environmental and genetic factors can increase your risk of developing type 1 diabetes.

Family members of people with type 1 diabetes may be eligible for autoantibody testing. Having autoantibodies puts you at a higher risk of developing type 1 diabetes.

Race and ethnicity can also put you at risk for developing type 2 diabetes. For unknown reasons, some people are at higher risk, including blacks, Hispanics, Native Americans, Africans, and Asians.

Prediabetes, type 2 diabetes, and gestational diabetes are common in people who are overweight or obese.

Symptom

Long-term complications of diabetes develop gradually. The longer diabetes persists and the less able you are to control your blood sugar, the higher your risk of complications. Ultimately, the complications of diabetes can be debilitating and life-threatening. In fact, prediabetes can lead to type 2 diabetes. Possible complications include:

Cardiovascular Disease

Diabetes significantly increases the risk of many heart diseases. These include coronary heart disease with chest pain (angina), heart attack, stroke, and narrowing of the arteries (atherosclerosis). If you have diabetes, you are more likely to develop heart disease and stroke. Nerve damage caused by diabetes (diabetic neuropathy). Consuming too much sugar can damage the walls of the small blood vessels (capillaries) that carry nutrients to your body, especially your legs. This may cause tingling, numbness, burning or pain, often starting in the toes and hands and spreading upward.

Damage to the organs involved in digestion can cause problems such as nausea, vomiting, diarrhea, and constipation. Erectile dysfunction can also occur in men. Kidney damage due to diabetes (diabetic nephropathy). The kidneys contain millions of glomeruli that help remove waste from the blood. Diabetes can damage this delicate information processing system. Eye damage due to diabetes (diabetic retinopathy). Diabetes can damage blood vessels in the eyes.

This can lead to blindness, foot injury, damage to the nerves in the feet and impaired blood circulation in the feet increases the risk of foot complications. The color and the condition of the mouth are also like that. Diabetes can make you prone to skin problems such as bacterial and fungal infections. Listen to the words of disobedience. Hearing loss is common in people with diabetes. Alzheimer's. Type 2 diabetes may increase your risk of developing dementia, such as Alzheimer's disease.

Depression related to diabetes

Symptoms of depression are common in people with type 1 and type 2 diabetes. Complications of Gestational Diabetes

Most women with gestational diabetes conceive healthy babies. However, if your blood sugar levels are not treated or controlled, problems can occur for you and your baby.

Gestational diabetes can cause complications in your baby, including:

Excessive growth

Excess glucose can cross the placenta. Excess glucose causes your baby's pancreas to produce more insulin. This can make labor difficult and sometimes require a caesarean section. Hypoglycemia. Babies born to mothers with gestational diabetes may have low blood sugar levels (hypoglycemia) shortly after birth.

This is because it produces more insulin on its own. Later, type 2 diabetes develops. Babies born to mothers with gestational diabetes have a higher risk of obesity and type 2 diabetes later in life. death. If gestational diabetes is left untreated, the baby may die before or soon after birth. Gestational diabetes can also cause complications in mothers, including:

Preeclampsia

Symptoms of this disease include high blood pressure, excess protein in the urine, and swelling of the legs and feet. Diabetes during pregnancy. If you had gestational diabetes during one pregnancy, you are more likely to develop it again during your next pregnancy. prevent

Type 1 diabetes cannot be prevented. However, making healthy lifestyle choices that help you manage prediabetes, type 2 diabetes, and gestational diabetes can also help prevent:

Eat Healthy

Focus on fruits, vegetables, and whole grains. Eat a variety of foods to avoid boredom. Get more physical activity. Try to get about 30 minutes of moderate aerobic exercise most days of the week. Otherwise, try getting at least 150 minutes of moderate aerobic exercise each week.

For example, take a brisk walk every day. If you can't exercise for long periods of time, try breaking it up into smaller activities throughout your day. Lose excess weight. If you are overweight, losing just 7% of your body weight can reduce your risk of diabetes.

For example, if you weigh 200 pounds (90.7 kg), losing 14 pounds (6.4 kg) will reduce your risk of developing diabetes. However, do not try to lose weight while pregnant.

Talk to your doctor about how much weight you can safely gain during pregnancy. To keep your weight at a healthy level, continue to change your eating and exercise habits. Consider these benefits of losing weight: A healthier heart, more energy, and higher self-esteem.

Medication may be an option. Oral diabetes medications, such as metformin (Glumezza, Fortamet, etc.), may reduce the risk of developing type 2 diabetes. However, a healthy lifestyle is important. If you have prediabetes, check your blood sugar at least once a year to make sure you do not have type 2 diabetes.

Foods To Eat When Diabetic

Vegetable

Vegetables are a food group that most of us don't eat enough of. It is rich in nutrients such as vitamins, minerals, and antioxidants. Vegetables are often divided into two types: non-starchy vegetables and starchy vegetables.

Starchy vegetables contain more carbohydrates, about 15 grams per half cup of cooked produce, so keep this in mind when planning your menu. Eat a variety of vegetables to get a variety of nutrients. Fresh vegetables are best. Frozen and canned foods are also good choices. It is inexpensive and may have a long shelf life. Check the sodium content.

low starch vegetables

Spinach, kale, kale, radish, mustard greens

pimento

carrot

vegetable

cauliflower

Brussels Sprouts

asparagus

Promise

onion

tomato

zucchini

garlic

mushroom

 okra

starchy vegetables

pumpkin

Winter squash (pumpkin, pumpkin, etc.)

jam

potato

 yucca

cassava

 but

 pea

fruit

If you have diabetes, fruits are a good choice. It contains many nutrients, including carbohydrates (about 15 grams per serving). Fruits also contain fiber, which helps lower blood sugar levels. Don't be afraid of frozen fruit. Typically harvested at the height of the growing season, they are just as nutritious as fresh fruit. Plus, since it's stored in the freezer, you don't have to worry about it spoiling quickly. If you have freezer space, buy in bulk when they are on sale. Frozen fruit is ideal for adding to smoothies or thawing with oatmeal or milk.

banana

yellow lemon

green lemon

plum

apricot

fishing

strawberry

Blueberries

grape

orange, tangerine

bean

Although it takes more time and skill to prepare, it costs a fraction of the price of many other protein-rich foods.

Using a pressure cooker rather than a pressure cooker can significantly reduce the time you spend in the kitchen. The price is reasonable even at the bank. One-third of a cup of baked beans contains about 15 grams of carbohydrates, as well as fiber, plant-based protein and other nutrients.

black beans

white beans

butter beans

pea

red bean

clean beans

bean

seed

If you have diabetes, you can also eat regular grains and other foods high in starch. Collect more than 50% of all seeds. And watch your intake. 1/3 cup of cooked nuts contains about 15 grams of carbohydrates. To add volume, add more bruising vegetables.

quinoa

barley

Pasta: Made from legumes (lentils, mung beans, black beans...), whole grains, other grains (quinoa, brown rice).

Bread (1 slice): Look for 100% whole wheat or 100% whole grain.

Virus

If possible, choose lean meat to reduce your saturated fat intake. Eat plenty of protein, including seafood, twice a week. Most of the animal proteins listed here contain 0 grams of carbohydrates. However, you should not consume too much protein. One serving contains 3 to 4 ounces of cooked meat. egg

Fish and other seafood, including shrimp, salmon, haddock, haddock, scallops, sardines, and tuna. Chicken (including chicken breast, chicken thighs, ground chicken, ground turkey)

Red meat such as beef, beef patties, flank steak, lean ground beef, tenderloin, etc.

Pork (including tenderloin, pork ribs, minced pork)

Dairy

Dairy products contain certain carbohydrates. A cup of milk contains about 12 grams, but dairy products also contain protein, calcium, and vitamin D. If you want to limit saturated fat, choose low-fat or low-fat dairy products. But the biggest thing to watch out for is sweetened dairy products such as yogurt and sweetened milk. This is because added sugar can cause it to contain a lot of carbohydrates. Instead, choose unsweetened yogurt or other dairy products and add fruit if desired. Compared to most dairy products, cheese is low in carbohydrates and high in protein and fat. milk

regular milk

white cheese

fruits and nuts

Fruits and nuts provide healthy fats and plant-based proteins with few carbohydrates in your diet. If possible, choose foods that are low in sodium or salt. Fruits and nuts make great snacks or toppings for oatmeal or salads.

almond

walnut

pecan

pistachio

peanut

chia seeds

flaxseed

hemp seeds

hazelnut

Food

10 Best Foods to Fight Diabetes

1. Cinnamon

This aromatic spice has been shown to lower cholesterol and keep blood sugar levels more stable. A 2019 study published in the International Journal of Dietetics found that participants who added 3 to 6 grams (about 1 to 2 teaspoons) of cinnamon to their daily diet had lower sugar levels. Blood is lower. small. Add cinnamon to your meals by adding it to smoothies, milk, oatmeal, or coffee. What are the other benefits of cinnamon? You can add flavor to your dishes without adding sugar or salt.

2. Fruit

Nuts are especially rich in polyunsaturated fat, which helps fight heart disease and improve blood sugar levels. These healthy fats have been shown to help prevent and slow the progression of diseases such as diabetes and heart disease. Almonds, pistachios, and pecans also contain these healthy fats. Fruits are low in carbohydrates, high in protein and fat, and are good for maintaining blood sugar levels. A little fruit goes a long way, so be careful about how much you consume. According to the USDA, 1/4 cup of shelled nuts contains 164 calories.

3. Oatmeal

Whole grains like oats are good for lowering blood sugar (adding them can reduce blood sugar spikes) and may help improve insulin sensitivity. Oats contain fiber in the form of beta-glucan, a type of soluble fiber that helps oats dissolve in water. Soluble fiber regulates blood sugar levels by slowing the absorption of carbohydrates from other foods.

In a 2019 pilot study published in the Journal of Experimental and Clinical Endocrinology and Diabetes, researchers gave participants about 3/4 cup of oatmeal per day for two days, which reduced their insulin needs over those two days. Interestingly, the study also found cinnamon in oatmeal, so combining oats and cinnamon may be a powerful combination to lower blood sugar.

Studies have shown that oats may help improve blood pressure, cholesterol levels, and fasting insulin levels.

4. Dairy products

Dairy products not only provide bone-strengthening calcium and vitamin D, but they are also a good source of protein to fight hunger. Milk, cheese, and yogurt are known to help stabilize blood sugar levels, and increasing your intake of these dairy products may reduce your risk of diabetes. Studies have shown that there is no need to consume low-fat dairy products.

A large analysis by researchers at Harvard University and Tufts University published in the journal PLOS Medicine in 2018 found that higher intake of full-fat dairy products (or whole-fat dairy products) was associated with a lower risk of obesity. Higher incidence of diabetes. It turns out they are relatives. Higher fat content makes you feel fuller, which reduces your tendency to crave sweets or high-carbohydrate snacks later. However, keep in mind that full-fat dairy products contain more calories than low-fat dairy products.

Therefore, you need to be careful about your intake. Whether you choose skim or whole milk, it's especially important to consider the amount of added sugar in flavored yogurts and dairy products. They can add significant calories in the form of simple carbohydrates.

5. Beans

Beans are high in fiber and protein, helping you feel full. Beans are also a good source of carbohydrates, containing about 20 grams of carbohydrates per half serving, according to the USDA. A 2020 review in the journal Nutrition found that beans may help reduce blood sugar and A1c levels in diabetics. Beans are inexpensive and extremely versatile. Add variety to salads and vegetable soups by adding different types of beans, such as black beans, pinto beans, chickpeas and cannellini beans.

6. Broccoli

Broccoli and other cruciferous vegetables such as kale, cauliflower and Brussels sprouts contain a compound called sulforaphane. According to a 2017 study published in the journal Science Translational Medicine, this anti-inflammatory compound helps control blood sugar levels and protect blood vessels from diabetes-related damage. Not only is broccoli low in calories and carbs (1 cup of cooked florets has just 55 calories and 11 g carbs, according to the U.S. Department of Agriculture), but it's also packed with nutrients like vitamin C and iron. Fill half your plate with these calming green vegetables.

7. Quinoa

This protein-rich whole grain is a great alternative to white pasta or white rice. According to the USDA, 1/2 cup of cooked quinoa contains 3 grams of fiber and 4 grams of protein. Rich in fiber and protein, quinoa digests slowly, keeping you full and preventing blood sugar spikes. Several studies, including a 2022 study published in the journal Nutrients, show that consuming quinoa reduces blood sugar levels after meals containing quinoa and may prevent the progression of prediabetes into type 2 diabetes. Quinoa is also a complete protein containing all 9 essential amino acids needed to build muscle, which is rare among plant-based protein sources.

8. Money

Garlic is one of the best sources of magnesium, which helps the body use insulin to absorb blood sugar and control blood sugar levels more effectively. A 2020 study published in the Journal of Nutrition found that women with polycystic ovary syndrome who took thylakoids, a substance found in vegetables, had significant reductions in weight, waist circumference, and blood insulin levels. It's done. Compared with placebo group after 12 weeks. This leafy vegetable is rich in vitamin K and folate, among many other important nutrients.

Additionally, according to the USDA, 2 cups of raw spinach provide only 2 grams of carbs and 14 calories. Enjoy your baby's raw vegetables in salads, add them to your morning smoothie, or blend them with garlic and olive oil for a nutritious treat.

9. Olive oil

This Mediterranean diet certainly ensures the success of diabetes treatment, especially thanks to its high content of monounsaturated fatty acids (MUFA). Several studies, including his 2017 review in the journal Nutrition & Diabetes, show that diets rich in MUFAs may improve blood sugar levels by reducing insulin resistance and increasing cell function. to help the body respond to insulin. It has proven useful for controlling values. With olive oil, you don't have to worry about fat.

Fats contain more calories per gram than carbohydrates, but they help keep you full, reduce blood sugar levels, and help your body absorb important nutrients like vitamins A and E.

10. Salmon

In addition to its high protein content, salmon is rich in omega-3 fatty acids, which can help maintain heart health by lowering blood pressure and improving cholesterol levels. Other fatty fish containing omega-3 fatty acids, such as tuna, mackerel and sardines, also provide this protective effect. This is important for diabetics who are also at risk. Cardiovascular disease may occur.

However, studies such as the 2020 Lipids in Health and Disease Report found that consuming fish oil did not improve blood sugar levels. . Make sure your diet includes omega-3s.

foods To Avoid

Knowing which foods to limit is just as important as knowing which foods to include in a diabetic's diet.

This is because many foods and drinks contain high amounts of carbohydrates and sugars, which can increase blood sugar levels. Other foods may have negative effects on heart health or cause weight gain. Foods to reduce or avoid if you have diabetes include:

1. Refined corn

Refined grains like white bread, pasta, and rice are high in carbohydrates but low in fiber, which can cause blood sugar levels to rise more quickly than whole grains. One research review found that whole grain rice was more effective than white rice at stabilizing blood sugar levels after a meal (32).

2. Sweet drinks

Sugary drinks like soda, sweet tea, and energy drinks not only lack essential nutrients, but they also have a high sugar content per serving, which can raise blood sugar levels.

3. Fried food

Fried foods are high in trans fats, a type of fat linked to an increased risk of heart disease. Additionally, fried foods such as french fries, nachos, and mozzarella sticks are often high in calories and may contribute to weight gain (33).

4. Origin

People with diabetes are often advised to limit their alcohol intake. This is because alcohol can increase the risk of hypoglycemia, especially if consumed on an empty stomach.

5. Breakfast Cereal

Most of these breakfast foods are high in sugar. Depending on the brand, one serving can contain as much sugar as a dessert. When purchasing cereal, read the nutritional information carefully and choose low-sugar varieties. Or, you can opt for oatmeal and add some natural sweetness with fresh fruit.

6. Candy

Each candy contains a lot of sugar. They often have a high glycemic index, which means your blood sugar levels are more likely to rise or fall after a meal.

7. Processed food

Processed foods like bacon, sausages, salami, and deli meats are high in sodium, preservatives, and other harmful compounds. Processed meats have also been linked to an increased risk of cardiovascular disease.

8. Fruit juice

You can drink pure fruit juice in moderation, but if you have diabetes, it is recommended to eat as much fruit as possible. This is because fruit juice contains all the carbohydrates and sugars found in fresh fruit, but none of the fiber needed to stabilize blood sugar levels.

10 Tips for Eating Healthy If You Have Diabetes

1. Choose Healthy Carbohydrates

All carbohydrates affect blood sugar levels. Choose healthy foods that contain carbohydrates and watch your portion sizes.

Here are some healthy sources of carbohydrates:

Whole grains such as brown rice, buckwheat, and whole oats.

Fruit

Vegetable

Legumes such as chickpeas, beans, and lentils.

Dairy products such as unsweetened yogurt and milk. At the same time, it is important to reduce your intake of low-fiber foods such as white bread, white rice, and highly processed grains. When in doubt, check food labels to find foods high in fiber.

2. Limit your salt intake.

Consuming too much salt increases your risk of high blood pressure and increases your risk of heart disease and stroke. And if you have diabetes, you are at risk for all of these diseases.

Limit your salt intake to a maximum of 6 grams (1 teaspoon) per day. Many packaged foods contain salt. So be sure to check food labels and choose foods that are low in salt. If you're cooking from scratch, be careful about your salt intake. You can also get creative and replace the salt with other herbs and spices to add flavor.

3. Reduce your intake of red and processed meat.

If you reduce your carbohydrate intake, you may need to eat more meat to feel full. However, it is not suitable for red meat or processed meat such as ham, bacon, sausage, beef, and lamb. All of these are linked to heart problems and disease. Switch to red or processed meat.

Legumes such as beans and lentils

Egg

Fish

Poultry, such as chicken and turkey

Unsalted fruit

Beans, peas and lentils are high in fiber and have little effect on blood sugar levels, making them a great alternative to red and processed meats and helping you feel full longer. Most people know that fish is healthy, but fatty fish like salmon and mackerel are even healthier. It is rich in substances called omega-3 oils, which help protect the heart. Eat two servings of oily fish per week.

4. Eat plenty of fruits and vegetables.

We know that eating fruits and vegetables is good for your health. It's always a good idea to eat a larger meal or snack when you're hungry. This will help you get the vitamins, minerals, and fiber you need every day to stay healthy.

You may be wondering if you should avoid fruits because they are high in sugar. My answer is no. All fruits are good for everyone, even if you have diabetes. This is different from added sugar (also called free sugar) found in chocolate, cookies, and cakes.

Choose whole fruit, as products like fruit juice may also contain added sugar. It can be fresh, frozen, dried, or canned (juice, not syrup). Additionally, it is better to eat it every day rather than a large amount at once.

5. Choose healthy fats

Fat is a source of energy and is essential to all of our diets. However, different types of fat have different health effects. Healthy fats are found in foods such as unsalted nuts, seeds, avocados, fatty fish, olive oil, canola oil, and sunflower oil. Some saturated fats can raise blood cholesterol and increase the risk of heart disease. These are mainly animal products and processed foods, such as:

Red meat and processed meat

Melted butter

Oil

Monkey oil

Cookies, cakes, pies, pastries. In general, it's a good idea to limit your oil use and use cooking, steaming, or grilling instead.

6. Reduce added sugar

We know that quitting sugar can be difficult at first. So small, practical steps are a good starting point for reducing your sugar intake. Start by swapping sugary drinks, energy drinks, and fruit juices for water, milk, unsweetened tea, or coffee.

Avoiding added sugar can help control blood sugar and weight. You can always try low-calorie or no-calorie sweeteners (also called artificial or sugar-free sweeteners) to reduce your intake. It may also help you lose weight in the short term if you don't replace it with other high-calorie foods and drinks. But in the long run, try to reduce the overall flavor of your diet.

7. Use your snacks wisely

If you need a snack, choose yogurt, unsalted fruit, nuts, seeds and vegetables instead of chips, cookies and chocolate. But be careful about the amount of food you eat. Helps maintain weight.

8. Dink Alcohol Sensibly

Alcohol is very high in calories. So, if you drink alcohol and are trying to lose weight, it may be a good idea to cut back on alcohol. Limit it to a maximum of 14 times a week.

If you take insulin or other diabetes medications, do not take this on an empty stomach. This is because alcohol can increase the risk of low blood sugar.

9. No need to worry about the so-called diabetes diet.

It is currently illegal to call a food a "diabetic food." That' because there's no evidence that these foods offer any significant benefits over a healthy diet. They also often contain the same amount of fat and calories as similar products and can also affect blood sugar levels. This food may also have a laxative effect.

10. Get minerals and vitamins from your diet.

There is no evidence that mineral and vitamin supplements help control diabetes. Therefore, you do not need to take supplements such as folic acid during pregnancy unless recommended by your healthcare team. Eating a variety of foods is a good way to get the nutrients you need. This is because some supplements may interfere with medication or worsen some cancer complications, such as kidney disease. Don't forget to move forward

Increased physical activity goes hand in hand with a healthier lifestyle. It also helps control diabetes and reduces the risk of heart disease. This is because the amount of glucose used by the muscles increases, allowing the body to use insulin more efficiently. Aim for at least 150 minutes of moderate exercise each week. This is any activity that increases heart rate, rapid breathing, and alertness. You can still talk and breathe a little. Plus, you don't have to do 150 minutes at a time. Break it down into 10 minutes a week, or 30 minutes five times a week.

Foods To Avoid When Diabetic

Treating diabetes requires a lot of attention and can sometimes be difficult. If you have diabetes, learn what foods to avoid to stay healthy and avoid blood sugar spikes. In fact, one of the most effective ways to combat diabetes is to eat a healthy, balanced diet. To help you better understand how to stabilize your blood sugar through diet, let's take a look at some of the most important foods to avoid if you have diabetes.

13 foods that help prevent diabetes

Many foods can be part of a sugar-free diet, but you don't have to follow a strict diet. However, people with diabetes should avoid or at least limit certain foods. To help you make healthier choices, here are 13 foods to avoid if you have diabetes.

1. Full-fat dairy products

Full-fat dairy products include cheese, ice cream, and whole milk. Although not suitable for moderate consumption, they often contain a lot of saturated fat. Eating too much saturated fat can raise your LDL (bad) cholesterol, increasing your risk of heart disease. Some studies also suggest that saturated fat may be linked to insulin resistance, a condition that worsens over time and is common in type 2 diabetes.

All of these behaviors should be avoided to reduce the severity of the addiction. It has a negative effect on insulin resistance.

Take the time to learn how to read nutrition labels and choose healthier alternatives instead of high-fat dairy products. Be careful not to choose options with added sugar to replace lost fat.

2. Trans fatty acids

Trans fatty acids are also foods to avoid if you have diabetes. Like saturated fat, trans fat has been linked to insulin resistance and increased levels of bad cholesterol. Trans fats can also cause weight gain and increase your risk of diabetes. Lastly, trans fats have been shown to have inflammatory effects that may increase the risk of diabetes-related complications. Trans fats can affect blood vessels, leading to high blood pressure and cardiovascular disease.

3. White Carbohydrates

White carbohydrates, known as "simple" carbohydrates, have little nutritional value. Refined carbohydrates have their fiber removed, making them easier for your body to digest. Although this looks promising, removing it quickly may cause blood sugar levels to rise quickly without providing any benefit to the body. Counting carbohydrates can help control blood sugar, but if you have diabetes, you should avoid white carbohydrates. Instead, add whole grains to your diet, which take longer to digest, provide long-lasting energy, and have a lower impact on blood sugar.

4. Fried Food

Fried foods are cooked using a lot of oil. This oil is composed almost entirely of saturated fatty acids, which are known to have negative effects on the treatment of diabetes. Unfortunately, frying reduces nutritional value and can also produce empty calories. Depending on the type of fried food you eat (such as french fries), you may be consuming a lot of sodium. Snacking here and there won't lower your blood sugar, but if you have diabetes, it's best to limit or avoid fried foods.

5. Alcohol

Alcohol has a negative effect on diabetes. You can drink it occasionally, but only in moderation. Also, avoid drinking too much and remember that you can have fun without drinking. If you are having trouble controlling your drinking, talk to your doctor and get professional help.

6. Processed Food

Processed meat is meat that has been treated with preservatives to extend its shelf life. Typically, this includes hot dogs, bacon, ham, hotdogs, etc. Processed meats are convenient, but they often contain high amounts of sodium, which can raise blood pressure. Diabetes increases your risk of heart disease, so you should control your sodium intake to further reduce your risk. Processed meats are also low in nutrients but high in calories, which is why many people call them 'empty calories.' It offers no direct health benefits and is therefore best avoided.

7. Fatty meat

You should also avoid meats high in fat if you have diabetes. These include pork or beef ribs, brisket, and various types of steak. Red meat has also been linked to an increased risk of heart disease and cancer, which affects people with diabetes. Instead, eat mainly lean proteins or lean red meat, such as sirloin steak.

8. Packaged Cookies and Cakes.

Packaged products are carefully processed and contain many additives. This is especially true for packaged breads, cookies and other baked goods. These foods tend to be high in fat but also contain simple carbohydrates. Unfortunately, simple carbohydrates can cause your blood sugar levels to rise quickly and dangerously. If you crave cookies or brownies while managing diabetes, look for sugar-free recipes online. Try these diabetic desserts that will satisfy even your sweet tooth.

9. Foods rich in sodium

Sodium has no direct effect on blood sugar levels, but it can increase blood pressure. Living with diabetes can increase your risk of many diabetes-related complications. Therefore, if you have diabetes, it is best to avoid foods high in sodium. Also, visit your doctor regularly, monitor your blood pressure, and make sure you are doing everything you can to minimize unnecessary risks.

10. Breakfast Cereals

Not all breakfast cereals are created equal. Some of them are healthy and rich in fiber, while others contain only sugar and refined carbohydrates. If you look at the nutrition label on your favorite childhood cereal, you'll see that sugar is the second or third ingredient. It is not good for treating diabetes. Consuming a lot of sugar in the morning increases your insulin levels and causes your blood sugar to spike early in the morning.

This can lead to increased drug addiction and a day full of twists and turns. Additionally, consuming too much sugar increases the risk of obesity, which has a negative impact on diabetes management.

11. Dried fruits

Dried fruits are good for your health, but you should avoid eating them if you have diabetes. Dried fruit often contains all the sugars of the whole fruit but comes in small pieces. This allows you to eat the sugar that some fruits contain right away without having to think about it. Instead, eat fresh fruit to satisfy your sweet tooth and get plenty of fiber.

12. Products containing added sugar

Although sugar does not directly cause type 2 diabetes, it can cause blood sugar levels to spike to dangerous levels. Unfortunately, sugar is added to many foods to improve taste. Always take the time to read nutrition labels and avoid foods with added sugar. This includes fruit juices, low-fat alternatives, and all processed foods. You may be surprised to learn that many packaged foods contain added sugar.

13. Carbonated And Energy Drinks

Lastly, almost all soft drinks and energy drinks contain sugar. Some "diet" drinks may contain sugar substitutes, but they are not necessarily safer than natural sugar. If you have diabetes, it is best to avoid these products and instead use flavored sparkling water or water infused with herbs or fresh orange.

Meal Plan

7 Day Diabetes Meal Plan

Controlling blood sugar levels is important to successfully overcome diabetes and prevent some complications. Eating healthy and maintaining a healthy diet can be helpful.

A healthy diet involves eating a variety of foods and helping you achieve or maintain a healthy weight.

The two 7-day meal plans included are perfect for people who are on a low-calorie diet and need a nutritional source for weight loss. One provides 1200 calories per day and the other provides 1600 calories per day. However, there is no one-size-fits-all plan. Ultimately, it is best to develop your own diet plan with the help of a doctor or nutritionist. prevent

Meal plans for diabetes help you track carbs and calories and introduce new nutritional ideas to make healthy eating more fun.

However, this eating plan may not provide enough calories for some people, including those who are very active, who are pregnant or breastfeeding, or who have certain medical conditions. Additionally, low-calorie diets may be more restrictive and make it more difficult to meet nutritional needs.

Careful planning is therefore essential. The plan below includes per-meal and daily carbohydrate intakes based on estimates from reliable USDA sources. This includes three meals a day, including snacks, all of which contain at least three servings of healthy, fiber-rich carbohydrates. You should consult your doctor or nutritionist to determine if the amounts listed below are appropriate for you. You can adjust as needed by changing portion sizes or adding snacks or meals.

Step By Step Guides

Diabetics can benefit from a healthy and varied diet that helps control blood sugar levels.

The evolution of this type of diet includes:

Balance Carbs, Protein and Fat to meet your nutritional goals

Measure the normal rate

Plan Ahead

With this in mind, the following steps will help you create a 7-day healthy eating plan. Stick to your daily calorie and carbohydrate goals.

Determine how much carbohydrates and other nutrients you should consume to achieve these goals.

Divide this amount into meals and snacks throughout the day. Find out where your favorite or familiar foods are and include them in your diet based on the information above.

Fill your daily calendar with deal lists and other resources from trusted sources. The side dish menu can change depending on the number of cabinets, making it easy to swap one type of food for another.

You can also group foods with the same fat and protein content into subcategories. Plan meals to maximize nutrient absorption, such as eating fried chicken one day and chicken cutlet the next.

Repeat this process every day of the week.

Monitor your blood sugar levels and normal weight daily to ensure your plan is producing the results you want.

Diet

Factors that influence the food choices of people with diabetes include:

Balance carbohydrate intake with activity level and use of insulin and other medications

Contains lots of fiber to help control blood sugar levels.

Limit highly processed carbohydrates and foods with added sugar

understand how food choices can affect complications of diabetes, such as high blood pressure

weight management

taking into account your individual treatment plan and the recommendations of your doctor or nutritionist

Combining the different methods below can be helpful when planning healthy meals.

Weight management

There appears to be a link between diabetes and obesity. Many people with diabetes may want to lose weight or avoid gaining weight.

One way to control your weight is to count calories. Your rcalories each day as a person depends on factors such as:

blood glucose concentration

activity level

height

sex

Specific plans to lose, gain or maintain weight

use insulin and other medications

favourite

finance

Different diet approaches can help people achieve and maintain a healthy weight, and not all of them involve counting calories. For example, the DASH diet focuses primarily on fruits, vegetables, whole grains, nuts and seeds, as well as low-fat or fat-free dairy products, poultry and fish. She advises people to avoid salt, sugar, unhealthy fats, red meat and processed carbohydrates.

The DASH diet is thought to improve blood pressure in people with hypertension, but research from reliable sources also shows that it may also help with weight loss and weight control. Your doctor or dietitian can give you additional advice about weight management.

Plate Method

It is important for people to consume the right amount of nutrients in their diet. The plate method uses an image of a standard 9-inch plate to help you visualize nutritional balance when planning your meals. Authoritative sources from the Centers for Disease Control and Prevention (CDC) recommend that the entire disc contain:

Made from 50% non-starchy vegetables

25% lean protein such as lentils, tofu, fish, lean chicken or turkey

25% fiber-rich carbohydrates like grains and legumes

If you need to increase your carbohydrate intake, you can add a small amount of fresh fruit or a glass of milk. Some oils are healthy and low in calories, while others are high in calories. These oils can be used in cooking and as a seasoning, but it is important to consume them in moderation. Consuming limited amounts of monounsaturated fats, such as olive oil, canola oil and avocados, will promote health, as will eating limited amounts of polyunsaturated fats, such as nuts and seeds, sesame and nuts, saturated fats found in coconut oil, animal fats and dairy products can increase cholesterol levels, a risk factor for cardiovascular disease.

Current dietary guidelines recommend:

45-65% of adults' calories come from carbohydrates

Less than 10% sugar

20 to 35% comes from fat, of which less than 10% comes from saturated fatty acids

10 to 35% comes from protein

You can ask your doctor if these instructions are right for you. Some people with diabetes need to reduce their carbohydrate intake to better control their blood sugar levels.

Carbohydrate Control

According to the National Institute of Diabetes and Digestive and Kidney Diseases, one way to control your blood sugar is to determine how many carbohydrates you eat each day and how they are distributed in your diet. A list of carbohydrate substitutes can help people decide how to "use" carbohydrates. Experts advise diabetics to avoid standard carbohydrates because each person's needs are different. The type of carbohydrate can also affect the amount of food a person can eat. Refined carbohydrates and sugars can quickly raise blood sugar levels without providing any nutritional benefit. Fiber, on the other hand, is digested slowly, helping to control weight and blood sugar levels. Current guidelines recommend a fiber intake of 25 to 38 grams per day for most adults, depending on age and gender. It's best to talk to your doctor about your calorie intake, how much food you need to eat, and how to distribute them throughout the day.

7-day diabetes meal plan

Medical Report by Jerlyn Jones, MS MPA RDN LD CLT, Nutrition - Written by Danielle Dresden - Updated May 15, 2023

Prevent

Step by step guide

Consideration

1,200 calorie plan

1,600 calorie plan

Limit fruit

Bring it all together

Final

Controlling blood sugar levels is key to living with diabetes successfully and avoiding some of its complications. Eating a healthy diet and maintaining a healthy diet can help. A healthy diet involves eating a variety of foods and helping you achieve or maintain a healthy weight.

In this article, he shares two 7-day meal plans that are suitable for those on a low-calorie diet and are a trusted source of weight loss support. One provides 1200 calories per day and the other provides 1600 calories per day.

However, there is no one-size-fits-all plan. Ultimately, it is best to develop your own diet plan with the help of a doctor or nutritionist.

PREVENTION

Meal plans for diabetes help you track carbs and calories and introduce new nutritional ideas to make healthy eating more fun.

However, this eating plan may not provide enough calories for some people, including those who are very active, who are pregnant or breastfeeding, or who have certain medical conditions. Additionally, low-calorie diets may be more restrictive and make it more difficult to meet nutritional needs. Careful planning is therefore essential. The plan below includes per-meal and daily carbohydrate intake based on estimates from reliable USDA sources.

This includes three meals a day, including snacks, with each meal containing at least three servings of healthy. fiber-rich carbohydrates.

You should consult your doctor or nutritionist to determine if the amounts below are right for you. You can adjust your serving size or add snacks or meals as needed.

Instructions step by step

Limit your intake of pasta, beans, and dried vegetables

Measuring portions allows you to accurately track your food.

Diabetics can benefit from a healthy and varied diet that helps control blood sugar levels.

The development of this type of food includes:

Balance Carbs, Protein and Fat to meet your nutritional goals

Measure the normal rate

Plan Ahead

With that in mind, the following steps will help you create a 7-day healthy meal plan for her.

Stick to your daily calorie and carb goals. Determine how many servings of carbohydrates and other food components will meet these goals. Divide this amount into meals and snacks throughout the day. Check the locations of your favorite and familiar foods and consider incorporating the above information into your meals. Fill your daily schedule with bargain listings and other resources from trusted sources.

The side dish menu can be swapped depending on the number of cabinets, making it easy to replace one type of food with another. You can also group foods with similar fat and protein content into subcategories.

Plan your meals to increase your nutritional intake, such as eating fried chicken one day and chicken fried steak the next. Monitor your daily blood sugar levels and your normal weight to see if your plan is delivering the results you want.

Food For Thought

Diet can help people with diabetes manage their disease. Vitaly Vodolsky/Shutterstock

Factors that affect the eating habits of people with diabetes include:

Balance carbohydrate intake, activity level, insulin consumption and other medications

Eat plenty of fiber to control blood sugar levels. reliable source

Limit your intake of highly processed carbohydrates and foods with added sugar

Understand how diet affects complications of diabetes such as high blood pressure

Weight Management

Taking into account your individual treatment plan and the recommendations of your doctor or nutritionist

Combining the different methods below will help you create a healthy diet.

weight management

There appears to be a link between diabetes and obesity. Many people with diabetes try to lose weight or avoid gaining weight.

One way to control your weight is to count your calories. The number of calories a person needs each day is determined by the following factors:

Blood sugar concentration

Activity level

Height

Sex

A specific plan to lose, gain, and maintain weight

Use of insulin and other medications.

Honey

A variety of diet methods can help you achieve and maintain a healthy weight, but not all diet methods involve counting calories.

For example, the DASH diet focuses primarily on fruits, vegetables, whole grains, nuts, and seeds, as well as low-fat or low-fat dairy products, poultry, and fish. She advises people to avoid salt, sugar, unhealthy fats, red meat and processed carbohydrates.

The DASH diet is thought to improve blood pressure in people with hypertension. However, studies from reliable sources have shown that it may help with weight loss and weight control. Your doctor or dietitian can give you additional advice about weight management.

Plate Method

Those using the disc method

The plate eating method helps you eat the right amount of each type of food. half point/shutterstock

It is important for people to consume the right amount of nutrients in their diet.

The plate method uses an image of a standard 9-inch plate to help you visualize nutritional balance when planning your meals. Authoritative sources from the Centers for Disease Control and Prevention (CDC) recommend that the entire disc contain:

Made from 50% non-starchy vegetables

25% lean protein such as lentils, tofu, fish, lean chicken or turkey

25% fiber-rich carbohydrates like grains and legumes

If you need to increase your carbohydrate intake, you can add a small amount of fresh fruit or a glass of milk. Some oils are healthy and low in calories, while others are high in calories. This oil can be used in cooking or as a seasoning, but it is important to consume it in moderation.

Consuming limited amounts of monounsaturated fats, such as olive oil, canola oil, and avocado oil, and limited amounts of polyunsaturated fats, such as nuts and seeds, promote health. Sesame seeds and nuts. maybe.

Saturated fats found in coconut oil, animal fats and dairy products can increase cholesterol levels, a risk factor for cardiovascular disease. Current dietary guidelines recommend:

45-65% of adults' calories come from carbohydrates

Less than 10% sugar

20 to 35% comes from fat, of which less than 10% comes from saturated fatty acids

10 to 35% comes from protein

You can ask your doctor if these instructions are right for you. Some people with diabetes need to reduce their carbohydrate intake to better control their blood sugar.

Carbohydrate control

According to the National Institute of Diabetes and Digestive and Kidney Diseases, one way to control blood sugar is to decide how many carbohydrates you eat each day and how they are distributed in your diet. The list of carb substitutions allows people to decide how to "use" their carbs.

Experts advise people with diabetes to avoid eating standard amounts of carbohydrates because each person's needs are different. The type of carbohydrate can also affect the amount of food a person can eat. Refined carbohydrates and sugars can quickly raise blood sugar levels without providing any nutritional benefit.

Fiber, on the other hand, is digested slowly and helps control weight and blood sugar levels. Current guidelines recommend that most adults consume 25 to 38 grams of fiber per day, depending on age and gender. It's best to talk to your doctor about your calorie intake, how much food you should eat, and how to distribute it throughout the day.

Glycemic Index

Foods with a high GI cause your blood sugar levels to rise quickly. These foods are heavily processed and contain sugar and calories. Low-calorie foods contain little or no carbohydrates or fiber, so the body does not absorb as much as processed carbohydrates.

Examples of carbohydrate-rich foods and their GI values are:

Low GI (score of 55 or less): 100% stone-ground whole grain bread, sweet potatoes with skin on, lots of fruit, whole grain oats.

Medium GI (56-69): oatmeal, brown rice, whole-grain flatbreads

High GI value (70 or more): white bread, red potatoes, candy, white rice, melon

1,200 calorie plan

The 1,200-calorie-a-day plan includes the following foods and snacks:

Monday

Breakfast: Spread a boiled egg and half a small avocado on a slice of Ezekiel bread and an orange. Total calories: 39.

Lunch: Mexican Bowl: 2/3 cup canned pinto beans, 1 cup chopped spinach, 1 cup chopped tomatoes, 1/4 chopped tomato, 1/4 green pepper, 1 ounce cheese. 1 tablespoon salsa.

Total Calories: 30 Snack: Eat 1 gram of baby carrots with 2 tablespoons of hummus. Total calories: 21.

Dinner: 1 cup cooked lentils, 2 ounces ground turkey, 1.5 cups vegetarian tomato sauce with garlic, mushrooms, greens, zucchini, and eggplant. Total calories: 35. Total calories per day: 125.

Tuesday

Breakfast: 3/4 cup blueberries, 1 cup cooked oatmeal, 1 ounce almonds, 1 teaspoon chia seeds.

Total calories: 34. Lunch: Salad: 1/2 cup green beans, 2 cups fresh vegetables, 2 ounces chicken breast, 1/2 small avocado, 1/2 cup cinnamon, 1/4 cup carrots, 2 tbsp.

Total calories: 52 calories. Snack: Add chopped small peaches to 1/3 cup of 2% cottage cheese. Total calories: 16 Dinner: Mediterranean couscous: 2/3 cup cooked whole grain couscous, 1/2 cup dried fruit, 4 sun-dried tomatoes, 5 chopped olives, 1/2 chopped cucumber, balsamic vinegar, 1 teaspoon fresh basil.Total calories: 38.

Total calories for the day: 140.

Wednesday.

Breakfast: Vegetable omelet with 3/4 cup blueberries, spinach, mushrooms, bell peppers, avocado, and 1/2 cup black beans. Total Calories: 34

Lunch: Sandwich: 2 slices 100% whole wheat, 1 tablespoon low-fat plain Greek yogurt, 1 tablespoon mustard, 2 cans marinated tuna with carrots, 1 tablespoon dill relish, 1 cup. Tomato slices, half a medium apple.

Total calories: 40.

Snack: 1 glass of unsweetened kefir. Total calories: 12 Dinner: 1/2 cup succotash, 1 teaspoon butter, 2 ounces pork tenderloin, 1 cup cooked asparagus, 1/2 cup fresh pineapple. Total calories: 34. Total calories per day: 120.

Thursday

Breakfast: Sweet Potato Toast: Top with 2 sweet potato slices, 30g goat cheese, spinach and 1 teaspoon boiling water.

Total calories: 44

Lunch: 2 ounces grilled chicken, 1 cup cauliflower florets, 1 tablespoon low-fat French dressing, 1 cup fresh strawberries. Total calories: 23.

Snack: Mix 1 cup of low-fat Greek yogurt with half a small banana. Total calories: 15 Dinner: 2/3 cup quinoa, 8 ounces soft tofu, 1 cup cooked bok choy, 1 cup steamed broccoli, 2 teaspoons olive oil, 1 kiwi.

Total calories: 44.

Total calories per day: 126.

Friday

Breakfast: 3 cups of oatmeal or high-fiber cereal, 1/2 cup of blueberries, and 1 cup of unsweetened almond milk. Total calories: 41.

Lunch: Salad: 1/4 cup tomatoes, 2 cups spinach, 1 ounce cheddar cheese, 1 ounce cottage cheese, 1 scrambled egg, 2 cups yogurt, 1/4 cup grapes, 1 pumpkin seed, 2 boiled green beans.

Total calories: 47.

Snack: 1 cup of celery and 1 tablespoon of peanut butter. Total calories: 6.

Dinner: 2 ounces salmon fillet, 1 medium baked potato, 1 teaspoon butter, 1.5 cups steamed asparagus. Total calories: 39.

Total calories per day: 133.

Saturday

Breakfast: 1 cup low-fat sweetened Greek yogurt with half a mashed banana, 1 cup strawberries, and 1 tablespoon chia seeds. Total calories: 32.

Lunch: Tacos: 2 tortillas, 1/3 cup cooked black beans, 1 ounce low-fat cheese, 2 tablespoons avocado, 1 cup coleslaw, salsa for dressing.

Total calories: 70.

Snack: 1 cherry tomato, 10 baby carrots, 2 tablespoons hummus.

Total calories: 14 Dinner: 1/2 roasted potato with skin removed, 2 ounces roast beef, 1 teaspoon butter, 1.5 cups steamed broccoli sprinkled with 1 teaspoon nutritional yeast, 3 to 4 cups whole strawberries.

Total calories: 41.

Total calories per day: 157.

Sunday

Breakfast: Chocolate Peanut Oatmeal: 1 cup cooked oatmeal, 1 tablespoon vegan chocolate or whey protein powder, 1 tablespoon peanut butter, and 1 tablespoon chia seeds. Total calories: 21 Lunch: 1 small bag of whole grain pita chips, 1/2 cup cucumber,

1/2 cup tomato, 1/2 cup lentils, 1/2 leafy greens, 2 salad dressings.

Total calories: 30.

Snack: Small grapefruit, 1 pound almonds. Total calories: 26. Dinner: 1/2 cup cooked radishes, 2 ounces cooked shrimp, 1 cup green beans, 1 teaspoon butter, 1 cup roasted radishes, 1 teaspoon balsamic vinegar.

Total calories: 39.

Total calories per day: 116.

1600 calorie plan

Monday

Breakfast: A slice of Ezekiel bread and an orange topped with a boiled egg and half a small avocado. Total calories: 39. Lunch: Mexican bowl: 1/3 cup brown rice, 2/3 cup refried beans, 1 cup chopped spinach, 1/4 cup chopped tomatoes, 1/4 cup green peppers, 1.5 ounces cheese, 1 tablespoon salsa. Total calories: 43.

Snack: 10g baby carrots and 2 tablespoons hummus. Total calories: 21.

Dinner: 1 cup cooked lentils, 2 ounces ground turkey, 1.5 cups vegetarian tomato sauce with garlic, mushrooms, greens, zucchini, and eggplant. Total calories: 35. Snack: 1 cup cucumber, 2 teaspoons tahini. Total calories: 3.

Total calories per day: 141.

Tuesday

Breakfast: 3/4 cup blueberries, 1 cup boiled oatmeal, 30 g almonds, 2 teaspoons chia seeds.

Total calories: 39 Lunch: Salad: 1/2 cup green beans, 2 cups fresh vegetables, 3 ounces grilled chicken breast, 1/2 small avocado, 1/2 cup sliced strawberries, quartered carrots, tablespoon French vinaigrette. 2 cups.

Total calories: 49.

Snack: A two-ton glass of cottage cheese with a small peach cut into three pieces. Total calories: 16.

Dinner: Mediterranean couscous: 2/3 cup cooked wheat couscous, 1/2 cup roasted eggplant, 4 sun-dried tomatoes, 5 giant olive slices, half a chopped cucumber, 1 tablespoon balsamic vinegar, fresh basil.

Total calories: 38.

Snack: 1 apple and 2 teaspoons almond butter. Total calories: 16.

Total calories per day: 158.

Wednesday

Breakfast: Vegetable omelet with 1 cup blueberries, 2 eggs, spinach, mushrooms, peppers, avocado, and 1/2 cup black beans. Total calories: 43. Lunch: Sandwich: 2 slices plain 100% whole wheat, 1 tablespoon low-fat Greek yogurt, 1 tablespoon mustard, 3 ounces marinated tuna with 4 cups chopped carrots, 1 tablespoon dill relish, 1 cup chopped tomatoes, half medium. apologize.

Total calories: 43.

Snack: 1 glass of unsweetened kefir.

Total calories: 12.

Dinner: 1/2 cup succotash, 1.5 ounces tortillas, 1 teaspoon butter, 3 ounces pork tenderloin, 1 cup cooked asparagus, 1/2 cup fresh pineapple. Total calories: 47.

Snack: 1 cup peanuts, 1 cup carrots. Total calories: 15.

Total calories per day: 160.

Thursday

Breakfast: Sweet Potato Toast: Top 2 sweet potatoes with 1 ounce goat cheese, spinach, and 1 tbsp. Total calories: 44.

Lunch: 3 oz roasted chicken, 1.5 cups cauliflower, 1 tablespoon vinaigrette, 1 cup fresh strawberries.

Total Calories: 23

Snack: Mix 1 cup low-fat Greek yogurt with half a small banana. Total calories: 15. Dinner: 2/3 cup quinoa, 8 ounces soft tofu, 1 cup cooked bok choy, 1 cup steamed broccoli, 2 teaspoons olive oil, 1 kiwi. Total calories: 44. Snack: 1 cup celery, 1.5 teaspoons peanut butter.

Total calories: 6.

Total calories per day: 132.

Friday

Breakfast: 1/3 cup raisins or other fiber-rich food, 1/2 cup blueberries, and 1 cup unsweetened almond milk. Total Calories: 41 Lunch: Salad: 1/4 cup tomatoes, 2 cups spinach, 1 ounce cheddar cheese, 1 chopped dried egg, 2 tablespoons yogurt dressing, 1/4 grapes, 1 pumpkin seed, 2 roasted chickpeas.

Total calories: 47.

Snack: 1 cup of celery and 1 tablespoon of peanut butter. Total calories: 6. Dinner: 3 ounces salmon fillet, 1 medium roasted potato, 1 teaspoon butter, 1.5 cups steamed asparagus. Total calories: 39. Snack: Half a cup of vegetable juice and 10 stuffed green olives.

Total calories: 24.

Total calories per day: 157.

Saturday

Breakfast: 1 cup low-fat sweetened Greek yogurt with half a mashed banana, 1 cup strawberries, and 1 tablespoon chia seeds.

Total calories: 32.

Lunch: Tacos: 2 tortillas, 1/3 cup cooked black beans, 1 ounce low-fat cheese, 4 tablespoons avocado, 1 cup coleslaw, salsa for dressing.

Total calories: 76. Snack: 1 cherry tomato, 10 baby carrots, 2 tablespoons hummus.

Total calories: 14.

Dinner: Half a baked potato with the skin removed, 2 ounces roast beef, 1 teaspoon butter, 1.5 cups steamed broccoli sprinkled with 1 teaspoon nutritional yeast, and 3 to 4 cups whole strawberries. Total calories: 48. Snack: Half an avocado dipped in hot sauce.

Total calories: 9.

Total calories per day: 179.

Sunday

Breakfast: Chocolate Peanut Oatmeal: 1 cup cooked oatmeal, 1 tablespoon vegan chocolate or whey protein powder, 1.5 tablespoons peanut butter, and 1 tablespoon chia seeds.

Total calories: 21.

Lunch: Small bag of pita chips, half a cucumber, half a tomato, half a cup boiled, half a green leaf, three tablespoons of vinaigrette.

Total calories: 30.

Snack: 1 medium apple, 1 oz pumpkin seeds. Total calories: 26.

Dinner: 85 g boiled shrimp, 1 cup peas, 1 teaspoon butter, half a cup boiled radish, 1 cup fried radish, 1 teaspoon balsamic vinegar.

Total calories: 39.

Snack: 16 pistachios, 1 cup jicama.

Total calories: 15.

Total calories per day: 131. Fruit only.

Fruits are superfoods and can be included in a balanced diet for people with diabetes. However, you should always consider the carbohydrate content of fruits and adjust your diet accordingly.

According to the American Diabetes Association, people should choose fresh, canned or frozen fruit. If possible, it's a good idea to look for products without added sugar. People can still enjoy dried fruit and 100 percent fruit juice in moderation, but they may not be as filling as whole fruit.

Some fruits may also have a high glycemic index, such as:

pineapple

ripe banana

Some dried fruits, such as dates

pumpkin

People can include them in a healthy diabetes diet, but experts recommend watching their intake to avoid spikes in blood sugar levels.

Recipes

10 Sweet Recipe Ideas Perfect for Diabetics

1. Low-carb Mediterranean broccoli salad

This salad recipe contains non-starchy vegetables such as broccoli, artichoke hearts, sun-dried tomatoes, and onions. These foods are high in fiber, which helps you feel full for longer. Olives and olive oil are rich in monounsaturated fatty acids, which help reduce the risk of heart disease, according to the American Heart Association (AHA). According to the Centers for Disease Control and Prevention (CDC), diabetes doubles the risk of heart disease, so it's important to prioritize monounsaturated fats in your diabetic diet. your way. Additionally, this salad's creamy dressing uses high-protein Greek sour cream (25.2 grams per cup) instead of low-fat mayonnaise (10.3 grams fat, 1.6 grams shortening saturation per tablespoon).

One serving of this recipe (1/8 of the total) from Fitness Nutrition Blog contains 182 calories, 14.7 grams (g) carbohydrates, 5.9 g protein, 12.4 g fat and 3.6 g fiber.

2. Fried Chicken with Vegetables

Crackers can be prepared simply by baking them. And this recipe includes plenty of diabetic-friendly vegetables, including carrots, broccoli, pumpkin, and green onions. Paulson said they also offer chicken as a lean protein option. The American Diabetes Association

(ADA) recommends choosing skinless chicken to lower fat and cholesterol levels. And instead of salt, Liz's Healthy Table chicken and vegetable dishes are packed with flavor with garlic, jalapenos, fresh ginger, lime, and low-sodium soy sauce.

According to the U.S. Food and Drug Administration (FDA), consuming too much sodium can increase blood pressure and increase the risk of heart disease. One serving of this product (1/4 of the full recipe) contains 220 calories, 11 g carbohydrates, 26 g protein, 3 g sugar, 3 g fiber, 9 g fat (1.5 g saturated fat) and 380 mg saturated fat. (mg) Sodium.

If you want to add more carbohydrates, serve brown rice instead of whole grain white rice. Paulson says eating whole grains can help prevent blood sugar spikes. The United States Department of Agriculture (USDA) estimates that a half-cup of brown rice adds 150 calories and 33 grams of carbohydrates to a recipe.

3. Vegetarian Lentil Tacos

Tacos on an empty stomach

Great Cuisine

Classy Cooking's meatless tacos are made with green lentils, vegetable broth, diced tomatoes, green peppers, yellow onions, garlic, coriander, lime, and various spices (cumin, chili powder, ancho chili powder, paprika, cayenne pepper). It combines many healthy ingredients including (red pepper). A study published in April 2018 in the Journal of Nutrition found that using legumes like lentils instead of traditional tacos like rice slows sugar digestion and lowers blood sugar levels.

Prices are likely to fall. One serving (1/9 of the total) contains 145 calories, 2 grams of fat, 23 grams of carbohydrates, 10 grams of fiber, 2 grams of sugar, and 8 grams of protein. Paulson recommends wrapping the filling in tortillas, whole grain tortillas, or large lettuce leaves.

4. Try healthy chickencho.

For the healthiest version of the popular Chinese takeout dish, try General Tso's Chicken recipe from the Plate. Made with a lean protein source (boneless chicken breast) and seasoned with a little corn, salt, and pepper. Then make a paste by adding peanut butter, dried walnuts, toasted sesame seeds and chopped parsley. According to the ADA, peanut butter is a good source of heart-healthy monounsaturated fats. Finish with ketchup, rice vinegar, hoisin sauce, a little brown sugar, and soy sauce. (Be sure to use a low-sodium version of the sauce or spice, especially since the recipe contains 718 mg of sodium).

One quarter of this recipe contains 207 calories, 10 grams of carbohydrates, 12 grams of protein, 12 grams of fat (2 grams saturated), and 7 grams of sugar. "To make it low-carb, serve it with roasted or steamed vegetables instead of white rice," says Paulson.

5. Finish the sandwich with chicken salad.

Enjoy the taste of a sandwich without the carbs and unhealthy fats. This burger from Diabetic Foodie uses a lettuce wrap instead of a bun and a lean protein like ground chicken or ground turkey instead of pork. It also contains plenty of pickled cucumbers, radishes, and carrots, making it a great meal for people with type 2 diabetes. When seasoning your burgers, be sure to use low-sodium soy sauce.

The burger contains 242 calories, 11 grams of fat (3 grams saturated), 11 grams of carbohydrates, 2 grams of fiber, 11 grams of sugar, 23 grams of protein, and 561 milligrams of sodium.

6. Lemon Garlic Salmon

According to the AHA, fatty fish like salmon used in this formula are good sources of omega-3 polyunsaturated fatty acids. If you have type 2 diabetes, eating foods containing omega-3 fatty acids can reduce your risk of diabetes-related complications, including heart disease and stroke. This recipe calls for grilling salmon with delicious and healthy ingredients: lemon, lemon zest, garlic, olive oil, and fresh parsley.

One serving of Salmon from Healthy Fitness Foods contains 294 calories, 9 grams of carbohydrates, 29 grams of protein, 17 grams of fat (2 grams saturated), 2 grams of fiber and 2 grams of sugar. . Eating fish with a salad or adding steamed vegetables like asparagus will provide better balance.

7. Summer pizza with tomatoes, zucchini and quinoa

"It all starts with a quinoa and hummus batter, which is packed with fiber, healthy fats and protein," says Paulson. Use more hummus in your dips and add healthy toppings. "This recipe includes vegetables that 1 always recommend for diabetics who want to enjoy pizza," says Paulson. She adds that using non-starchy vegetables like pumpkin or tomatoes can add flavor, fiber, vitamins and minerals without overloading your diet with carbohydrates.

One serving (1/12th of the recipe) contains 150 calories, 13 grams of carbohydrates, 4 grams of protein, 10 grams of fat (1 gram saturated), 3 grams of fiber, and 1 gram of sugar.

8. Mexican Chopped Salad

This chopped salad from Café Sucre Farine contains a variety of non-starchy vegetables, including romaine lettuce, peppers, onions, jicama, zucchini, and tomatoes. It also contains black beans, which are rich in protein and fiber, which help keep you full (15.8 grams of protein and 18.1 grams of fiber per cup for the low-sodium variety).

Make your own scones and make our Homemade Honey Lemon Dressing recipe to see how much sodium and oil you're consuming. One-eighth of this recipe contains 228 calories, 8 grams of fat (1 gram saturated), 35 grams of carbohydrates, 10 grams of sugar, 5 grams of protein, and 7 grams of fiber. For more protein, add grilled chicken or fish.

9. Mediterranean salmon skewers

Erhardt's Grilled Salmon Skewers are delicious and healthy. Combine omega-3 rich fish fillets and non-starchy vegetables such as pumpkin, grape tomatoes, and red onions with dried spices, olive oil, and lemon. . Skewer and grill lean proteins and vegetables for a quick, healthy meal for diabetes. One serving (1/4 of the full recipe) contains 316 calories, 20.7 grams of fat (2.8 grams saturated), 4.3 grams of carbohydrates, 30.4 grams of protein, 1.2 grams of fiber, and 2.2 grams of sugar. Optional: Grilled meat skewers with tzatziki sauce.

10. Low-carb zucchini lasagna.

Paulson says traditional lasagna is high in calories, carbohydrates and saturated fat, making it unsuitable for people with type 2 diabetes. But this version from Diabetes Strong uses zucchini instead of pasta, which helps cut down on carbs and calories without sacrificing flavor. He added that pumpkin is used in many dishes. For example, a medium-sized pumpkin contains 35 grams of vitamin C, making it an excellent source of the nutrient.

Previous research has shown that many people with type 2 diabetes may be deficient in this antioxidant in their blood, possibly due to high levels of oxidative stress caused by abnormal blood sugar production. Paulson says this recipe uses 1/2 cup of lean ground beef and cheese to cut down on saturated fat. One quarter of this recipe contains 244 calories, 12.3 grams of carbohydrates, 30.4 grams of protein, 7.9 grams of fat (3.5 grams saturated), 6.3 grams of sugar, and 3.6 grams of carbohydrates.

Conclusion

Diabetes is a slowly developing disease with no cure. However, with proper knowledge and timely treatment, complications can be reduced. The three main complications are   blindness, kidney damage, and heart attack. It is important to closely monitor a patient's blood sugar levels to prevent complications. One of the problems with over-regulating blood sugar is that such efforts can lead to hypoglycemia, which can lead to greater complications as blood sugar levels rise.

Researchers are exploring other ways to treat diabetes. The purpose is to provide an overview of the current state of diabetes research. Diabetes is one of the most challenging research topics of the new millennium, and he wants to encourage new researchers to take up this challenge.

Diabetes is a public health problem that affected approximately 80 million people worldwide in 1990. This number is expected to double by 2000. In the United States alone, approximately 12 million people have diabetes, and this number is increasing every year. Cardiovascular disease accounts for most of the morbidity and mortality associated with diabetes.

In 1987, in the United States, more than 1 million diabetic patients with coronary artery disease or coronary artery disease as the main diagnosis were hospitalized, and more than 100,000 died. Mortality after acute myocardial infarction in patients with non-insulin-dependent diabetes mellitus (NIDDM) has been shown to be two-fold higher than in non-diabetic patients with similar infarction. They   also found that the age-adjusted mortality rate from cardiovascular disease in patients with diabetes was eight times higher than in non-diabetic patients, primarily due to the increased incidence of coronary heart disease. It has been reported to be an independent risk factor for vascular disease.

We also look at risk factors such as cholesterol levels, blood pressure, and smoking.